CASE HISTORY TAKING FOR OSTEOPATHS

with a touch of Differential Diagnosis

CASE HISTORY TAKING FOR OSTEOPATHS

*with a touch of
Differential Diagnosis*

by

T A Rulten BSc (Hons) Ost PGCE

ISBN 9798843245733

This book is dedicated to the amazing
students at the
European School of Osteopathy,
who bring joy to my life every Friday.

This book may never have materialized without the help and
support of some fabulous people:

Amy and Janet
Thank you so much for proofreading my work, and for your
invaluable suggestions and corrections.

Tim
Thank you for your osteopathic help, insight and support.

Barry
I'm so grateful for your graphic design wizardry.

Katherine
Thank you for your suggestions, endless support,
encouragement and love.

Contents

Introduction

In 1992, I decided to stop fixing computers and start fixing people instead. I left the security of my job at IBM, the world's biggest computer company at the time, and spent nearly two years travelling around the Greek islands and Africa. I returned to spend four years studying at the European School of Osteopathy. Since then, I have worked as an osteopath in private practice, and as a clinic tutor and lecturer at the European School of Osteopathy.

When I was studying osteopathy, I was frustrated by the lack of textbooks covering case history taking. Some medical textbooks would include a small section on history taking, but it often seemed to be a token gesture and was certainly not specific to the role of a physical therapist. Yet case history taking is the bedrock of any consultation. So, years later, when I was teaching Case History Taking and Differential Diagnosis, I wrote my own little booklet entitled *A brief guide to Case History Taking*. Students found it very useful, so I decided to revise and expand it, and along the way, include some help with differential diagnosis and basic hints and tips to help all physical therapists get the most from their consultations.

I hope you find this book helpful and enjoyable.

Terry Rulten

Who is this book for?

This book is aimed primarily at the student practitioner, whether they are studying osteopathy, chiropractic, physiotherapy or any other physical therapy. In addition, I hope experienced practitioners will benefit from a refresher in the art of case history taking.

What is a case history?

A case history is a record of the patient's experiences, not only of their current complaint for which help is being sought, but of their health, life, work and family situation. It details clinical findings, diagnoses and treatment, and records the patient's progress.

The case history is a legal document. It may be used as evidence in cases of litigation or insurance claims. It should be completed contemporaneously (at the time of the consultation), not later when the details have faded into the mists of time.

Why do we take a case history?

When I first started writing this book, I happened to watch a programme on TV about a girl who has 'medical vision' – the ability to look at someone and instantly 'see' what is wrong with them. Unfortunately, most of us are not blessed with this ability, and need to resort to more conventional means of diagnosing a problem. Once we have a diagnosis, we can implement an appropriate treatment and management plan.

Please note that I will use the term 'diagnosis', but in most cases, what we have in reality is a 'working hypothesis'. We work out what we think is wrong with our patient based on the information we obtain from the consultation, testing and examination, and we use our knowledge and experience to come up with a working hypothesis, or working diagnosis. This may change and be refined depending on how our patient progresses throughout their course of treatment.

When a patient first consults us, they could have virtually anything wrong with them. There are not enough hours in the day to examine and test for all possible problems and pathologies. We need to gather information to enable us to discount as much as we can, leaving us with the smallest number of possible diagnoses – the process of differential diagnosis. We then formulate an examination plan to test our hypotheses and ideally end up with a single working hypothesis. We can then develop and agree with the patient a suitable treatment and management plan.

What does a working diagnosis consist of?

A system that has always worked well for me is one where I strive to identify four things:

1. The tissue causing pain.
    This may be a muscle, ligament, joint capsule, disc, visceral organ etc, or even a combination of several. If we understand which tissue is causing the pain, we can choose the most appropriate techniques and management plan to help our patient. If we do not identify the correct tissue, we may use an inappropriate technique or management plan and fail to help our patient, or even make their condition worse.

2. Aetiology.
    What caused the injury? Was it a specific trauma? Was it due to a particular activity, lifestyle or situation? If we understand what caused the injury or condition, we can help the patient find a way to prevent it happening again.

3. Predisposing factors.
   What predisposed the patient to this particular injury? Is it maybe their exercise or work situation? Is it an existing medical, musculoskeletal or mental health condition? For example, a patient with a frozen shoulder may have an increased thoracic kyphosis which has compromised the shoulder mechanics, and made them more susceptible to a frozen shoulder.

4. Maintaining factors.
   What is maintaining the patient's injury? What is stopping them from getting better? For example, if your patient has a simple muscle strain, they should recover within a couple of weeks or so. If they haven't, you need to understand what is hindering their recovery. It may simply be that they have continued to over-exercise, so the muscle hasn't had a chance to recover. There may be other factors: their vitality may be low due to other health issues, they may have work or home stress, they may have poor nutrition or any number of factors which have reduced their ability to fully recover. I often find myself explaining to patients that it's like having a set of scales. On one side are things making you better: the body's own healing capacity, treatment, medication etc., and on the other side are the things hindering recovery: your other health issues, diet, stress etc. I frequently tell patients that our treatment is aimed at tipping the balance towards improved health. Please note that some maintaining factors are often the same as the predisposing factors.

Often in practice, a patient will arrive having sustained an injury — low back pain for instance, and they'll say something like 'all I did was bend down to take my shoes off'. Clearly, a person with reasonably good health should be able to take their shoes off without injuring themselves. So, in a case like this, we have to determine what predisposed them to this injury? What health and life factors have led them to be like this? My aim is always not just to help the patient to recover from their injury, but to enjoy better health than they had *before* the injury.

By understanding what caused the injury, what is maintaining it and what the predisposing and maintaining factors are, we can be truly holistic in our treatment and management of our patients. We can work to help heal the tissues causing pain, and we can help prevent a recurrence by addressing the predisposing and maintaining factors. Our management plan may include direct treatment, prescription of exercises, advice on work or home life, referral to another specialist and more. In doing so, we achieve much more than just helping them overcome an injury, we can help them to be the very best that they can be.

Differential diagnosis

Although this is a book on case history taking, it's impossible to cover the subject without a sprinkling of differential diagnosis (DD). The two are inextricably linked. In your early days as a student, you may be focusing on gathering information when taking a case, then analysing it to form your DD. But with knowledge and practice, you'll be able to tailor your case history taking, such that you will be formulating a DD 'in flight' while taking the case. This will enable you to ask certain questions to confirm or deny your various hypotheses.

All teaching establishments by necessity teach a course by dividing the training program into individual subjects: anatomy, pathology, physiology etc. It's probably the best way, but it causes our brains to compartmentalise the knowledge. This is good when you're sitting an exam. In a pathology exam for example, your brain will load up the 'pathology' module and away you go. *Academically*, you're in good shape. The issue in a clinical setting is that a patient doesn't come to the clinic saying 'I've got a pathology problem'. They might say 'I have a shoulder problem'. So, during the consultation, your brain will need to draw on knowledge from all the 'modules' in your brain, for information on what may be causing, or be a factor in, your patient's problem: anatomy, pathology, orthopedics, physiology and much more.

So, I'll give you a tip! Start to build up a knowledge base – either a folder or electronically, which has sections for each area of the body: neck, T spine, lower back, knee, hip etc., and for each region, build up aspects from anatomy, pathology, orthopedics etc., that are clinically relevant to that region. Not the in-depth, exam-passing type knowledge, but things like what pathologies can cause pain in that area, who gets them, what predisposes them to it, what are the other symptoms? What anatomical structures may be involved? What would the pain patterns be? Are there any congenital, inflammatory, neurological, neoplastic, traumatic, degenerative, referred, vascular, functional or metabolic causes? If you can get this *clinical* knowledge base in your head, your brain will fast access it while you're taking the case, giving you the best chance of formulating a fabulous DD.

Top-class academic knowledge is good, but we need top-class clinical knowledge to be able to do the best for our patients!

Now let's go back to case history taking:

Where do you start?

Put yourself in your new patient's shoes. What will they be thinking about on the way to see you? It is likely they will have thought through and rehearsed what they plan to say to you. They may not have seen a practitioner before, and be apprehensive about any number of things: What will you be like? Will you be able to work out what is wrong with them? Will you be able to help them? Will they have to undress? Will the treatment hurt? These and many other questions may be running through your patient's mind. It is your job to put them at ease and provide an atmosphere and environment that will allow effective case history taking.

Make sure that your room is set up correctly. Think about the positioning of chairs for you, your patient and anyone accompanying them. In a student clinic setting, you may have observers. There is nothing worse than having the patient cowering in the corner, with you and a host of observers across the other side of the room all staring and taking notes. Position the chairs to allow you to face the patient within a comfortable distance, while at the same time being able to take notes (using a table or the couch for example). Any observers may be best placed to the side.

Remember how important first impressions are. Greet the patient in a professional, friendly way. Explain who you are and ask them to come along to the consulting room. Even at this early stage, you should be starting the process of differential diagnosis. You will hopefully have observed the sex of your patient, which will rule in or out a significant number of pathologies straight away. Their age, physical appearance and demeanor will provide more clues, as will your observations of the way they move.

Small talk is a great thing. It puts the patient at ease and starts to build a rapport. Have a chat about the weather or anything you want. By the time you reach the consulting room, you should have broken the ice and be ready to take the history.

Many years ago, when I worked in the IT industry, we used a phrase 'bridge to business'. This was when the small talk changed to the business in hand. Make your patient comfortable and explain exactly what will happen. Explain to them how you are going to ask them about the problem they have come to see you about, and how you will ask about their past medical history and health in general. You need to explain that you will be asking them to undress as appropriate and that you will examine them to see what is wrong. In a teaching clinic setting, explain that you will need to discuss their case with a tutor, and that the tutor may come into the room at some time. You must check that the patient is happy with what you have told them and give them a chance to voice any concerns. They may want a chaperone, for example.

Gaining consent

It is essential that you gain your patient's informed consent. *In-formed* consent means the patient has been given all the information they require about what will happen during the session in order to decide whether or not to consent to it. At the start, this may refer to the initial consultation and the session in general, but will at some point refer to the examination and the possible need to undress and be physically examined. When discussing treatment and management options, you will need to explain possible risks and benefits.

I cannot emphasise enough the importance of effective communication between you and your patient in this area. Most patient complaints arise from miscommunication: something has happened that they did not expect. As a practitioner, you must constantly be aware of how your patient is feeling throughout the consultation. Look for clues; body language for example, as to how they are finding the whole experience. If you sense something is not right, then bring it up. It's fine to say something like 'I sense you're not completely comfortable. Is everything OK?' It gives them an opportunity to point out a misunderstanding, or an issue they have, and therefore allows you to resolve the issue there and then.

Your patient may dwell on something that happened during the consultation, and be unhappy about it, or they may talk to a family member who might suggest something was not right and this may lead to a complaint. Often, when patients have lodged a complaint with a governing body, the practitioner has commented that they 'sensed something was not right at the time, but didn't know what'. If they had raised it at the time with the patient, the issue could have been resolved straight away, and a whole lot of stress averted.

Taking the history

So, let's check: you have created a good impression, you look pro-fessional, have greeted the patient professionally, engaged in some friendly chit-chat, made them feel at home in your warm and airy consulting room and gained their permission to proceed. Now we need to get on with finding out what is wrong with them!

Taking a case history is having a conversation; a structured conver-sation. It's a two-way exchange of information. Like any conversa-tion, no two are the same. Every single consultation you have throughout your career will be different from any other. However, the format may be very similar in most consultations. You must have a framework or system to work by, that ensures that all rele-vant information is gathered and understood in a reasonable peri-od of time. This will enable you to develop a differential diagnosis and formulate a plan of examination, which will lead you to a diag-nosis and then a treatment and management plan. What is the tis-sue causing pain? What has caused the injury? What are the pre-disposing and maintaining factors? All these questions must be an-swered. The system we use in osteopathy is similar, but not the same as that used in mainstream medicine.

Understand that there is no pre-formatted list of questions that automatically follow one after another. If this were the case, we would simply hand the patient a questionnaire to fill out while they are waiting to see us. Our questioning should be logical and sys-tematic, but the questions we ask, and their order and depth, will be governed by the patient's responses. You need to be able to think on your feet and adapt the questioning as appropriate. It may be a shock, but we need to apply intelligence and common sense throughout the interview. In time, history taking will be instinctive; you will develop your own style that suits your personality and your patients. However, whatever your style, you must get the required information.

Time management

Always keep in mind the following responsibilities:

- Your patient expects you to apply 100% of your knowledge, skill and effort within the allotted time to find out what is wrong with them, and to treat them effectively.
- You will (hopefully) have a full list of patients one after the other expecting to be seen on time.
- You must always work safely.

The only way to reconcile all the above is by working efficiently. You must have the background knowledge and skill, and be able to apply it in a clinical setting. Taking the case history well is vital to your success. Practice alone will enable you to work quickly, safely and effectively. With time you will learn to identify the areas key to the case in hand which require extensive questioning and those areas which are of less relevance, but may swallow up time. This supplementary information may be gathered during treatment if need be.

The case history is divided into four main sections:

1. The presenting complaint (what the patient has primarily consulted you about).

2. Past medical history.

3. Systemic and general health.

4. A record of diagnosis, management plan, treatment and progress.

Our aim is to build a detailed picture of the patient's overall health: how it is now, how it has been in the past and how it progresses throughout a course of treatment.

These four sections can be further divided as follows:

Presenting complaint:

- Details of the presenting complaint.

- GP.

- Medication.

Systemic and General Health:

- Cardiovascular system.

- Respiratory system.

- Gastrointestinal system.

- Genitourinary system.

- Gynaecological system.

- Nervous system.

Family history.

Diet.

Allergies.

Exercise.

Social situation.

Past medical history:

- Accidents.

- Illnesses.

- Operations.

Impact.

Expectations.

Record of diagnosis, management plan, treatment and progress.

SOAP

Along with most healthcare professions, we use SOAP as a basis for the way we work – not just to keep us squeaky clean – it's an acronym:

Subjective
Objective
Assessment
Plan

The **Subjective** part is the story the patient tells you: the initial case history. Like any good detective, we use this information to identify the 'likely suspects'. We start the process of differential diagnosis – we narrow down the number of possible diagnoses which may be causing the patient's present problem. Once we have a list of possibilities, we can formulate an appropriate plan of examination and testing to differentiate between these possibilities.

The information gathered during our examination provides the **Objective** evidence. Using this evidence – the facts we have gathered – we arrive at our **Assessment** (diagnosis or working hypothesis). This enables us to implement a treatment and management **Plan**.

Note: this procedure (SOAP) is carried out every time you see your patient. They tell you how they have been since the last treatment (Subjective), you re-examine (Objective), and you reassess (Assessment) and review your treatment (Plan).

The presenting complaint

Please note that throughout this book, I will suggest questions to ask, and will generally word them in a way that I use in practice. It suits me, my personality, and the patients I see. However, you must find your own wording, and a style that suits you. For example, at this stage I might say:

'What's the problem you've come to see me about today?' Or *'How can I help you today?'*

Remember, you must find your own words to ask the same thing. I'm not trying to tell you exactly what to say.

As far as the patient is concerned, the presenting complaint is the reason for them coming to see you and the most important part of the consultation. There are a number of standard questions that you may ask that will help you to gather all the information necessary to form a working diagnosis.

In healthcare, as in other areas of work, acronyms are often used to help us remember things. When I was training to be an osteopath back in 1994, the standard questions regarding the presenting complaint were known as 'the ten points of pain'. It's a catchy title, and although the word pain is in the title, the same questions are used for any presenting complaint, even if it isn't pain. More recently, there has been a move to encourage osteopaths to use a similar set of questions to those used in mainstream medicine. One advantage of this is that a snappy acronym can be used to remember the points: SOCRATES. Personally, I feel we can remember the questions without an acronym, and the old system was better in that it generates more detail. It's no big deal, so long as you can gain all the information you need.

I have listed the questions associated with SOCRATES alongside the similar questions from the ten points of pain.

Site	Location
Onset	Onset
Character	Nature
Radiation	Radiation/referral
Associations	Associated symptoms
Time course	Progression
Exacerbating / relieving factors	Aggravating / relieving factors
Severity	Included in nature
	Daily pattern
	Duration
	Previous

Each of these questions is merely an opening enquiry. We ask follow-up questions based on the patient's responses until we have gathered enough information to allow us to narrow down the number of conditions the patient may be suffering from. This is the process of differential diagnosis. For example, we may know at the outset that the patient is suffering from right shoulder pain. This may be due to any number of conditions, such as; muscle strain, ligament sprain, adhesive capsulitis, dislocation, visceral referral, fracture and many more. We need to narrow down the number of possibilities in order to reduce the extent of our examination and testing. If you have narrowed down the number of possibilities to one, two or maybe three conditions, you only need to examine and test for these few possibilities to find out which is the correct diagnosis. Testing for everything possible is not being thorough, it is poor practice. If your case history has failed to exclude a raft of possible conditions, you will have to test for them all. You may spend so long examining and testing, you have no time to treat. This will not help with your patient's satisfaction.

In most cases, your patient will have already thought about what they are going to tell you. They will almost have a script planned. A nice open question such as 'How can I help you today?' will encourage them to start to tell their story. Some patients will instantly launch into a long and detailed account of their problem, and will often include a lot of information that is of little or no relevance to the case in hand. Others may be far less talkative, and will need some coaxing to get them to open up. It takes practice and skill to judge when and how to interrupt the patient's flow, as well as how to encourage them to open up and tell you the full story. I will come back to this later.

The 'ten points of pain' / SOCRATES

As stated previously, the process of taking a case history is not a rigid set of questions and answers. It is a professional, structured conversation, which will meander through various aspects of the case depending on the responses to the questions you ask, the situation in hand, and your personal style. The points are listed below in a certain order, but the order you ask the questions will vary with each case, dependent on the flow of responses. In most cases, I would suggest starting with the location of the pain.

Location / Site

It is important that you understand early on exactly where the pain is. Just asking 'where is the pain?' is often not good enough. You will be surprised how often a patient will talk of, say, 'shoulder pain' or 'hip pain' or 'coccyx pain', but when you ask them to point to exactly where the pain is, it is not where you expect. So go ahead and ask them. For example, you might say 'Can you point to exactly where you experience your shoulder pain'. Make sure you understand the extent of the pain. Is the painful area a small point of 'spot tenderness' or is it spread over a large area? Get the patient to map out exactly how far the pain spreads. I like to get up and ask the patient if I can touch the area, partly to confirm exactly where the pain is experienced, and partly to see if this initial gentle touch will elicit pain.

Why is it so important to accurately locate the area of pain?

Remember, we are trying to identify the tissue causing pain. Part of your brain should be visualising the anatomical structures associated with the painful area, both deep and superficial. At first, this may be a conscious thing, but in time, you will be doing this subconsciously. In doing so, you can start to add flesh to the bones of a hypothesis. By keeping in mind the tissues which may be causing the pain at the location identified, you can modify and refine your questioning to confirm or discount your theories as the consultation progresses.

In addition, your mind should also be thinking of structures that may refer pain to the area under investigation. How are you going to differentiate between a local injury causing pain, and pain referred to the area from another structure? Read on.

Radiations / Referral

Radicular pain and referred pain are different things, but what the two terms have in common, is that pain is perceived in an area away from the tissue causing the pain.

It's an over simplification, but basically, radicular pain is generally due to the irritation of a nerve root, and therefore the pain follows the dermatome for that spinal level. The pain is generally sharp and shooting, and may be accompanied by pins and needles (parasthesia) and/or numbness, and may cause a degree of muscle weakness in any muscles served by that spinal nerve.

For example, if there is a disc bulge at L5/S1, it may impinge the L5 and/or S1 nerve root. This may cause sharp, shooting pain over the buttock, posterior thigh, lateral lower leg, foot and toes. In addition, there may be numbness in the foot and toes, and weakness in foot dorsiflexion (foot drop).

Referred pain generally originates from deep structures such as a visceral organ or joint capsule. The mechanism for pain referral is different from that of radicular pain, in that the pain is generally experienced somatically in an area which shares its innervation with that of the organ or joint capsule. The pain is usually dull and diffuse.

For example, an inflamed gall bladder may cause irritation to the phrenic nerve, which originates at C3, 4 and 5. The brain does not perceive pain from the gall bladder; instead, it perceives it somatically over the C3, 4 and 5 dermatomes, typically over the right shoulder.

I mentioned earlier the process of differential diagnosis: the use of information to rule in and rule out what could be causing the patient's symptoms. Well, this process starts right now.

Let's take as an example the case of a patient with right shoulder pain. There is a myriad of possible causes, but let's just look at three: a rotator cuff injury, referred pain from a facet joint in the neck, and referred pain from the gall bladder. Differentiating between these is relatively easy: a rotator cuff injury will give increased pain on shoulder movement, the facet problem will give pain on neck movement, and the gall bladder pain will not be affected by any joint movement, but will be related to when the patient is processing fatty food they have been eating.

We need to know what type of pain the patient is experiencing, and how bad it is. The way a patient describes their pain, will again, give us a clue to the tissue causing pain. Certain descriptions are suggestive, but not diagnostic of certain tissue injuries. At the end of this section is a table linking types of pain to tissues. Remember though, these descriptions are suggestive, not proof

Open questions such as 'How would you describe your pain?', and 'What type of pain is it?' are a good start. Your patient might respond straight away with 'It's like a knife' or 'It's an ache', for example. Sometimes though, when patients are asked to describe their pain, they have difficulty finding the right word. You may sit there waiting for some time while the patient struggles to come up with a suitable description, so occasionally it is appropriate to help the patient by using a 'menu' question. For example, 'Would you say it's sharp, dull, burning, or stabbing, for instance?'

Please note: while menu questions are useful and appropriate at times, the options you include must be of the same type. So, dull, sharp, stabbing are all types of pain, and are therefore OK when asking for pain descriptors, but later when we are asking about general health, for example, we would not ask something like 'Do you have any headache, weight loss, chest pain, dizziness etc', because these are questions relating to different systems. We would ask each question individually and wait for an answer.

As well as the type of pain, it is very useful to know how severe it is. 'How bad is the pain?' is good, but is very subjective. We can add a degree of objectivity by getting the patient to rate their pain out of 10. 'On a scale of 0 to 10, how bad is your pain, where 0 is no pain, and 10 is the worst pain you can imagine?' Get them to rate the pain when it's at its best, and at its worst. Some injuries may cause no pain for much of the time, but significant pain on a sudden movement: joint instability, for example. Some injuries, e.g. a strained muscle, may give a continuous background ache due to local inflammation, and increased pain on muscle contraction. You can see how the information you gather starts to point to certain injuries, tissues and processes. As well as helping us understand the cause, rating the amount of pain will give us a benchmark against which we measure progress over the course of treatment.

Take care if your patient describes their pain as 'constant'. You need to know if their pain is truly constant. By constant, we mean that the pain is there at all times day and night, unchanged by movement, activity or position. If this is the case, it is a 'red flag', a sign of likely pathology. So, if a patient tells me they have constant pain, I may ask 'So, do you mean you have the same pain, day and night no matter what you do?' or 'Do you mean there's always some background pain, but it's worse on certain movements or activities?' If this is the case, it's not so concerning.

Pain descriptors and associated structures / causes

Type of pain	Possible structure / cause
Cramping, dull, aching	Muscle
Sharp, shooting	Nerve
Deep, nagging	Bone, pathology
Sharp, severe, intolerable	Fracture
Throbbing, diffuse	Vascular

Duration

When your patient has the pain, how long does it last? By this I mean, do they get a sudden twinge, whereby the pain suddenly comes on, and quickly goes? Or does the pain come on and stay for some time? Are they ever completely pain free? This can give you an insight as to the process or mechanism of their injury. Sudden pain, relieving quickly may suggest joint instability, for example. If there is inflammation, the pain will not suddenly come on and then quickly go.

Question your patient closely to find out when and how the problem occurred. Be thorough and detailed in your questioning. We want to know when the pain came on, and more importantly, what caused it.

The patient may be very specific: 'It came on last Saturday, I lifted a plant pot', for example. Even so, we need more information: was their back OK before the lift? Did they feel the pain immediately, or did it come on later or even the next day? How did they lift the pot? If we can understand the mechanism of the activity, we can visualise the areas of the body, and the structures being put under load, which will enable us to ask specific questions to identify the nature of the injury in terms of the tissue causing pain and any physiological process going on such as inflammation.

Often, the patient is less specific. For example, they may say their pain came on sometime last month, but they have no idea what caused it. It's important to explore all possibilities here in order to test for pathology. In most cases of musculoskeletal injury, there will be a physical cause. If they say they can't think of any cause, maybe ask if they remember if it came on during the day, or did they wake with the pain, for example? If they woke with it, they might think they slept awkwardly. In most cases though, where the pain was first experienced on waking, it's because of something they did the day before. They may have sustained a minor strain or sprain and not noticed much at the time, but overnight, inflammation has built up and caused pain on waking. You will know that overnight, we produce less of our own natural anti-inflammatories, and so inflammation tends to get worse at night, causing us stiffness and pain in the morning. So, in this case, question them closely on what they were doing in the days before waking up in pain.

If they say the pain just came on during a day, ask them in detail what they were doing in the run-up to the pain becoming apparent. This may give you an insight into the mechanism of injury, or the process taking place. Is there anything that might explain their injury? Were they doing anything new, or outside their usual pattern of activity?

Gradual onset of pain without any reason, especially if it's getting worse, and not altered much by change of position or activity may be a sign of pathology. Later we will discuss systemic and general health screening.

Associated symptoms

Some injuries have particular associated symptoms which give clues to the true nature of the problem. Generally, we do not ask leading questions. We could ask 'Are there any symptoms associated with your back pain / neck pain / calf pain etc.?' However, the patient may not fully understand what you mean. Here we may need to be quite specific in our questioning. For example, for a patient with low back pain: is there a problem or change to their bowel or bladder habit? (Evidence of a somato-visceral or viscero-somatic problem). A patient with neck pain: do they have headache? (Evidence of cervicogenic headache or pathology). A patient with knee pain: is there any clicking or giving way? (Evidence of meniscal problems). Of course, there are many more associated symptoms for many more primary complaints. I have only listed a few examples to make a point.

Check with the patient on the timing of these associated symptoms. In the case of neck pain and headache, for example, does the headache come on only when there is neck pain? Does the patient have headache without neck pain sometimes, and vice versa? Was the original onset of both symptoms at roughly the same time? This line of questioning will help you decide if one symptom is a direct result of the other, or whether one predisposes or exacerbates the other, or if there are two unrelated issues.

I'm sure you know how good our bodies are at compensating and adapting following an injury. If, say, a patient has a sprained ankle, they will automatically adapt and compensate to take some of the load off the injured ankle. This could lead to pain elsewhere, possibly the lower back and/or neck. In this case you would expect the pain due to compensation to come on days or maybe weeks after the original injury. Technically, this isn't an associated symptom, but is of course related to the primary issue.

By understanding the extent of any associated symptoms and their timing relative to the presenting complaint, we can further refine our differential diagnosis.

Daily pattern

Some injuries and pathologies produce symptoms which vary through the day in characteristic patterns. For example, some disc lesions may cause minimal pain when the patient first wakes, but once they are weight bearing and active their pain increases. Someone with degenerative joint disease may be very stiff on waking, which eases after moving about, but gets worse again later in the day after work. Severe stiffness in the morning lasting more than an hour may be suggestive of an inflammatory condition. Ask your patient if there are times throughout the day when they tend to be better or worse. Ask them what they are like when they first wake. Ask yourself if their pattern matches any 'typical' patterns.

Of course, there may be no consistent daily pattern. This in itself can be very telling. Is it the case that their pain only comes on during certain activities? If so, you can work out which tissues may be under load

What makes it worse? *Exactly* what aggravates the pain? Remember, you are trying to gather evidence to suggest the tissue causing pain. So if, for example, a patient says that their pain is made worse when driving their car, what is it about driving that makes them worse? Is it when they turn the steering wheel? Is it when they change gear? Is it purely the seated position? Is it when they turn to reverse? Are they actually in pain while driving, or is it after a long drive when they get out of the car? Each situation will be more or less suggestive of what is causing their problem, and will add another piece to the jigsaw. As physical therapists, with our knowledge of mechanics, we should be expert at identifying which tissues are under strain at any given time.

TIP: When you are planning your examination, bear in mind what your patient has told you about the positions they find painful. Many times in the teaching clinic I have had a student explain, for example, how their patient is acute and can't stand straight, and then go on to say how they intend to have their patient lie prone on the couch. This is unacceptable.

Given the location of the pain, you were able to visualise the structures and tissues that may be causing the pain, and the structures and tissues that may refer pain to that area. Your knowledge and training should enable you to understand how these various tissues may be stressed, and therefore produce pain. You may ask questions like: 'What makes the pain worse?' Or 'Are there any activities, movements or positions that aggravate your pain?' If you understand what makes the pain worse, you can move closer to identifying the tissue causing pain.

So, when do certain tissues cause pain? Let's take a look at some.

Muscles

In order to understand muscular pain, it may be useful to review the various 'muscle states'. Muscles are there to cause movement of a joint by contracting and relaxing. If we exercise a muscle, it may become hypertrophied – we build muscle bulk. If we have a prolonged period of inactivity, our muscles will atrophy – they get smaller, or waste. These are 'normal' muscle states.

If a muscle is overworked, tissue damage within the muscle may occur – a muscle strain which will cause an inflammatory response.

Although muscles need to work to stay healthy, skeletal muscles are not meant to stay contracted for long periods of time. If they do, they can become fibrotic. They become less elastic and fatigue or strain more easily. This is one reason why poor posture may lead to some spinal muscles becoming dry and fibrotic, and achy from being habitually held contracted.

If our brain detects pain signals, it will often cause a muscle contracture over the painful area in order to protect it. Unfortunately, sometimes the pain from this muscle spasm is worse than the pain from the underlying injury. So be careful: if you decide your patient has pain due to a tight muscle, it's no good just releasing the muscle. You have to work out why the brain is telling it to be tight. Is it a protective contracture, or part of an adaptive pattern, or are the muscles fibrotic and ischemic due to chronic hypertonicity?

In general, muscle pain is aching in nature, made worse when contracted or stretched. In the case of a strain, there may be a background ache much of the time, made worse on contraction. Plus, on examination, there will be pain on palpation, pain on active movement, but minimal pain on passive movement.

Although we are talking about case history taking, it's worth mentioning here that when you are examining your patient, it is essential that you ask them exactly where the pain is while you are examining them. For example, if your patient has low back pain, then on active movements, if they side-bend to the right and they say it's painful, we need to know exactly where. If the pain is on the right, we are thinking of the structures being compressed, but if the pain is on the left, we are considering the structures being stretched. For example, a left quadratus lumborum strain may produce pain on the left as it is stretched on right side-bending, and possibly more pain as it contracts to help the patient straighten.

Tendons

As you know, tendons attach the muscles to the bones either side of a joint, and are therefore under load when the muscle contracts, or is stretched. The mechanism for a tendon strain is very similar to that of a muscle strain – if the muscle and tendon are overloaded, tissue damage may occur. We can differentiate between a muscle strain and a tendon strain on examination using palpation. Simply put, if the tender area is over a tendon, that's where the problem is, if it's over the muscle belly, then you have a muscle strain.

Ligaments

Ligaments are there to limit the range of movement of a joint, and so will be damaged or produce pain when the joint is taken beyond its natural range of motion, or when the ligament is under load for too long. A common example is an ankle sprain. The ankle joint is less stable when plantar flexed, making it vulnerable to an eversion sprain. The ankle turns over into eversion putting the lateral collateral ligaments under load. This may cause pain of short duration while under load, or if the load is great, and damage occurs, pain may last for weeks while the ligament heals. In addition, when the ankle turns over, the brain will try to limit the potential damage by contracting muscles to prevent over eversion. This could result in a muscle strain as well as a ligament sprain.

Another example is when we sit slumped in a chair for too long. If there's a gap between one's lower back and the chair, then the spine will be flexed. The ligaments between the vertebrae will limit the amount of flexion, and after a time, will start to signal that it's time to move by starting to produce pain – usually an ache. Interestingly, the erector spinae muscles will also be working to reduce the flexion, and after a time will become fatigued and generate pain – also an ache. This will occur sooner, if the muscles are dry and fibrotic from being held in high tone over long periods of time.

Joint capsules

Joint capsules form an envelope around each synovial joint to keep the synovial fluid in the joint space. Together with the accompanying ligaments and tendons, the capsule provides joint stability. Joint capsules are highly innervated, and are therefore very pain sensitive, particularly when they are stretched or 'nipped'. One common condition where this is very evident is in adhesive capsulitis of the shoulder, or 'frozen shoulder'. The joint capsule becomes inflamed, and can shrink, and is particularly painful on internal and external rotation of the glenohumeral joint, because this motion causes maximum stretch of the capsule. Therefore, in practice, the patient may say they can't brush their hair, or do up their bra, for instance. Another common capsule involvement you will see is facet joint problems in the spine. In some facet joint injuries, the joint will become hypertrophied – the joint capsule will swell. This of course will cause the capsule to be stretched, thereby causing pain. Imagine the effects on the capsule on various spinal movements: in forward flexion, the capsule will be progressively stretched, causing pain – often an ache getting worse towards the end of range of movement. On extension though, the capsule may be 'nipped', which will give immediate intense pain. In the case of the lumbar spine, this may be one reason why some patients adopt a flexed posture, or hold their backside slightly tucked under. In the cervical spine, they tend to stand with their neck slightly flexed. Most acute spinal facet joint injuries are unilateral and so may cause a degree of side-bending away from the painful side in addition to flexion, as the patient tries to avoid approximating the joint surfaces.

Intervertebral discs

In order to diagnose a disc injury, we must first understand the various types of disc lesions, and the pain patterns they produce. So, let's look at what happens to discs.

A normal healthy disc will have a jelly-like nucleus surrounded by a tough annulus which will allow movement between two vertebrae, as well as providing a degree of cushioning and shock absorption. The movement is controlled by the facet joints.

Degenerative disc disease: Over time, the nucleus will dry out somewhat, which reduces its flexibility. The disc will also become thinner. The problem with this is that the size of the lateral foramen is related to the thickness of the disc. As the disc gets thinner, the two vertebrae approximate thereby narrowing the lateral foramen, which may cause lateral stenosis. This process is most commonly age related, and may combine with osteophytic growth, which may further reduce the space available for the exiting spinal nerve to function, causing radicular symptoms.

Bear this in mind during the case history and examination: side-bending towards the narrowing would most likely make the symptoms worse, side-bending away, may relieve the symptoms. But nothing is certain! There could be a case where side-bending away from the painful side would stretch the nerve root over an osteophyte, causing radicular symptoms. It's useful to also understand that changes in one structure will affect the structure and function of others. When it comes to disc degeneration for example, as the disc degenerates, the centre of weight bearing moves posteriorly, causing the facet joints to bear some of the load, as well as the disc. The function of the facet joints is to guide and control movement, not to bear

load, so this will inevitably lead to dysfunction, compensation, adaptation and pain.

Disc prolapse: The annulus is a very tough structure made up of layers of cartilage with fibres arranged in each layer to give strength and mobility. However, the disc has weak spots at the postero-lateral aspects. This can allow the pressure of the nucleus to cause the disc to bulge – a disc prolapse. Nerve fibres may detect the stretch on the annulus and refer pain to the lower back if the disc is a lumbar disc or the neck if it's a cervical disc. (Disc prolapses are rare in the thoracic spine). Another consequence of a prolapse is that the bulge takes up space, and as there is no spare space anywhere in the body, something will be compressed. As the weak part of the disc is around the area where the spinal nerves exit the spinal canal, a disc bulge can result in nerve root impingement which may lead to pain, parasthesia, numbness and/or muscle weakness. If there is a large central prolapse in the lumbar spine, cauda equina may occur, which of course is a medical emergency.

In the case of a disc bulge, there is minimal inflammation, so the pain will be caused by the stretching of the annulus referring pain to the back or neck, but it's likely to be a mild or moderate ache. The symptoms to the leg, however, may well be quite significant; usually radiating pain over a dermatomal area. There may also be parasthesia, numbness and/or muscle weakness dependent on the nature of the impingement. Symptoms are often made worse on forward flexion and sitting.

Disc herniation: The annulus can become so weakened that it splits. Once this happens, the nucleus can migrate through the annulus. This is problematic for two main reasons: firstly, the herniated disc material will take up space, and as with a disc bulge, may well cause nerve impingement, and so radicular symptoms. Secondly, the herniated nucleus will be seen as a 'foreign object' and will prompt a significant inflammatory response, which will of course, cause significant pain – not only in the back or neck, but also in a radicular pattern if the inflammation irritates a nerve root.

Bursae

Bursae are little fluid-filled sacs which sit where muscles or tendons slide across bone. They provide an almost friction-less surface for the tendons to ride over. They are lined with a synovial membrane which secretes synovial fluid. Repetitive movement and excessive pressure may cause a bursa to become inflamed – bursitis – and therefore pain-ful and swollen. Pain will be quite local and tender when pressure is applied. Patients will find it painful on active movement when the muscle contracts and the tendon rubs on the bursa. If there is a muscle strain, or a tendon strain or bursitis, all will cause pain on the associated active movement. You can differentiate between the three by palpating to identify exactly where the painful structure is.

Be aware that it is rare for only one tissue to cause all the pain. This is one reason why some practitioners are not happy with the 'tissue causing pain' form of diagnosis. It may be too local and reductionist. However, it's a start, and we can broaden the diagnosis to include the wider pic-ture. For example, in the case of a spinal facet joint injury as mentioned above, the facet joint itself will produce a pain pattern typical of that injury, but whenever there is pain, the body will want to protect itself. This often takes the form of contraction of the muscles overlying the af-fected area, which in turn will produce muscular pain. There may be local inflammation which will cause pain. In some injuries, nerves may be irritated or impinged, causing local and radicular pain. And of course, compensatory pat-terns and postural adaptations may take place, putting other structures under load, and therefore pain.

Back to the ten points of pain / SOCRATES:

In the same way that knowing what makes the patient's pain worse helps us to understand the nature of the injury, so does understanding what reduces the pain.

Is there anything you can do that reduces the pain? This is a nice specific question that will encourage the patient to provide a specific answer, such as 'Yes, if I hold myself slightly bent forward', or 'If I don't put weight on my right leg', or 'Yes, applying heat helps', or 'Yes, I'm not in any pain while I'm sitting still'. It helps us understand the mechanism or process causing the pain, by knowing what reduces it. If we ask 'What makes the pain better?', the patient sometimes thinks we are asking what cures the overall condition, and they say 'nothing', so be specific in your questioning. As well as 'Is there anything you can do to reduce the pain?' I might ask 'Is there any position or activity that reduces the pain?'

Progression

The way our patient's symptoms have progressed since onset tells us much about the type of problem they have. Find out how your patient was, immediately after the incident (assuming there was an obvious cause of the injury), how the pain progressed later that day and over time since then. In some cases, it is helpful to draw a small pain / time graph. By understanding how their condition has progressed over time, you will be able to rule in, as well as rule out, various possible diagnoses. If there are associated symptoms, when did these occur? Try to build up as detailed a picture of how their condition has progressed as you can. Then, ask yourself if their pattern suggests any typical mechanisms of injury and recovery, compensation or pathology.

I mentioned above that the progression may help you to rule in, as well as rule out, certain conditions. One example is a patient you suspect may have a disc herniation. If they tell you the pain was very bad on day one (8/10) and very much better on day two (3/10), then this makes your hypothesis very unlikely. A true disc herniation will not resolve itself so quickly. You may think a patient has a muscle strain, but if the pain has persisted after, say, two months, it makes it unlikely. A simple muscle strain would have resolved itself, unless of course there are factors maintaining the injury.

Consider a patient with acute pain after lifting, easing somewhat after a few hours and continuing to ease over the next few days. Contrast this against someone who has pain of gradual onset for no good reason and getting progressively worse. The former is more suggestive of a mechanical strain, the latter of pathology. I know – I make it sound easy. Of course, in real life, things are not quite so obvious.

If your patient's condition has been getting worse, look for possible reasons: have they continued to do the very thing that caused their injury? Are there other health problems hindering recovery? Steadily worsening symptoms must be seen as a sign of pathology, especially if there was no clear onset. However, if there are good reasons to explain their poor recovery, the patient's problem may well be purely musculoskeletal. Please note though: always err on the side of caution!

Previous

Has the patient had a similar problem in the past? This can be a good question for several reasons. If the answer is yes, when did they first have the problem? How long did it last? What did they do about it? How many episodes have they had and when? Did they receive treatment – if so, what? Were they given a diagnosis? Have they had x-ray investigations or scans of the area in question? If so, what did they reveal? Although you cannot assume automatically that they have the same problem now, you will have an insight into any underlying dysfunction or weakness they may have. You may understand how well they will respond to treatment, and what type of treatment suits them best, based on their response to past treatment. If they have not had a similar problem before, you can reflect on why they have it now. What are the predisposing factors for their present predicament?

GP

Has the patient consulted their GP or other health professional regarding their present complaint? If so, what was the diagnosis? What tests were carried out? What action has been taken? If they have seen another healthcare professional, did they make a diagnosis? What was it? What treatment did they carry out? Did it help? This will give you an insight into what has helped and what has not, and so will inform your treatment and management plan.

It is usually at this point when I ask my patient a question like 'Have you taken any medication for your pain?' If they have taken medication for their presenting complaint, be sure to ask for details. We want to know what medication, the dosage, and when they have taken it. Also, is it helping? By knowing the type and amount of medication, and the effects it's had, we can form a view of the nature and severity of the injury.

Medication

You need to know what medication your patient is taking for the following reasons:

- Safety: It may contraindicate certain examinations or techniques.
  For example: Anticoagulants will contraindicate high velocity thrusts (HVTs). Long-term steroid use may predispose to osteoporosis and therefore contraindicate HVTs.

- The patient's presenting complaint may relate to a side effect of their medication.
- Your examination findings may be skewed by medication – analgesics for example.

Please note: when I say medication, I mean prescription medication, over the counter medication and supplements. So, what are they taking, and what dose? For how long and is it helping? Think about how relevant your patient's medication is to their condition.

Some practitioners will wait until they are moving on to the patient's general health before asking about their medication. My own preference is to ask at the end of the presenting complaint section. I might ask 'Have you taken any medication to help with your neck pain?' And of course, if they say yes, I'll get all the details. It then gives me a nice smooth transition into their general health. I might say something like 'Are you taking any medication for anything else?' They might answer something like 'Yes, I'm taking tablets for my blood pressure.' I can then ask them to tell me all about their blood pressure issues, and then 'How's your health otherwise? Do you have any other ongoing medical conditions you are aware of?' And before we know it, we're smoothly into the patient's general health.

Review so far

The case history process is like putting together a jigsaw puzzle. Each piece builds a picture of what is wrong with your patient: the tissue causing pain, the aetiology of the injury and the predisposing and maintaining factors. It should also build a 'big picture' placing the patient's health issue in context with their general health and life situation. The location, onset, nature and spread of pain are key to diagnosis, as are the other 'points of pain'. You are looking for factors that increase or reduce the likelihood of a range of diagnoses that may be present in this patient.

As a student, you may well be expected to justify your hypothesis by pointing to aspects of the case that support it. For example: 'The patient has most likely suffered a disc injury – a disc bulge. This is supported by the nature and location of the pain (acute low back pain with sharp pain radiating to the posterior thigh and lateral foot made worse on forward flexion), the daily pattern (better on waking but worse on weight bearing as the day goes on), and the traumatic onset (twisting while lifting a heavy sack). In addition, the patient is in the right age range (20 to 40 years).'

In the same way, you should be able to use aspects of the case to rule out certain hypotheses. For example: 'It is unlikely the patient has a disc herniation as he is 70 years old, his low back pain is a dull ache with no radiating pain and he has early morning stiffness easing on movement.'

This justification process is not limited to student life. Every time you take a case history in practice for the rest of your career, you should be going through the same process, but with yourself, instead of a tutor or examiner. This will raise the likelihood of you formulating the best hypothesis.

Systemic review

We must assess the patient's systemic health for the following reasons:

- We are primary healthcare practitioners. As such we have a duty to assess the general health of our patients and give appropriate advice.
- Your patient may have a systemic condition causing their presenting complaint.
- Your patient may have a systemic condition which has predisposed and/or maintained their presenting complaint, and may influence their recovery.

- Your patient's systemic health may influence your choice of treatment approach and technique. Indeed, they may have a systemic condition which contraindicates all or some physical therapy. They may even have a condition which requires urgent medical care.

Let me take a little detour here and ask a question: how will you know if a patient is suffering from a pathology or systemic condition? Here's another: if an elephant entered the room now, how would you recognise it? This may seem like a daft question, but let's go through it anyway. Of course, the answer is that your brain would compare the sight, sound, smell etc. with information it holds in the 'elephant' section of your brain. If this area were empty, you would not recognise what it was that was trampling you underfoot!

Likewise, how can you identify the tissue causing pain if you are not familiar with the relative anatomical structures and how they are put under load, and the types of pain they produce? Without a good anatomical knowledge base you will struggle.

How will you know if your patient is suffering from, say, bowel cancer if you do not know about bowel cancer? Do you know who gets it, the common age of onset, signs and symptoms etc.? Without a good knowledge of pathology and physiology you may be unsafe.

We generally focus on the major systems of the body: the cardiovascular system, the respiratory system, the genitourinary system, the gynaecological system, the gastrointestinal system, and the nervous system. For you to be able to question a patient intelligently, you must have knowledge of pathologies relating to each of these systems and an understanding of their symptoms. As a tip, I would suggest you make sure you are familiar with five or six of the common symptoms of failure of each system, and formulate questions accordingly.

Of course, it is not good enough to merely know the symptoms; you must know what questions to ask and practice asking them. It is all well and good knowing that dyspnoea may be a symptom of heart disease, but what do you actually say to the patient? Practice turning symptoms into questions phrased in common everyday language.

When we carry out a systemic review, we ask appropriate questions based on the case in hand, to assess the patient's systemic health. There is no set list of questions to ask. You and you alone must decide how extensive your questioning should be, based on the information gathered so far and your observations. In some cases, you may choose to conduct a 'basic screen' of their systemic health. In others, a thorough in-depth investigation will be indicated. Let's take a couple of examples:

1.   Your patient is a 24-year-old female aerobics instructor. She complains of a sprained ankle which she sustained two days ago when she tripped during a class. She is generally very healthy and has no history of significant ill health.

In this case, you may argue that a minimal systemic review is indicated such as: How is your health generally? Do you have any change to your bowel or bladder habit? Do you have any chest pain? Do you get out of breath when you would not expect to? Have you had any problems or change to your periods? Do you regularly suffer from headaches? Is your weight stable or changing?

2.   You have a patient complaining of low back pain around the right QL area. He describes it as a dull ache which is not affected by any particular movements or activities. Onset was gradual over the past week for no obvious reason.

We know that pain unaffected by movement is not suggestive of a mechanical or musculoskeletal injury. What other systems may be involved? Could the patient's pain be due to a gastrointestinal or genitourinary problem?

In this case your questioning would be more extensive. In addition to your basic screen, you might also ask questions such as: do you have any problems or change to your bladder habit? Do you have pain on urination? Have you noticed any blood in your urine? Have you felt an increased temperature or fever? Any problems or change to your bowel habit? Have you been constipated lately, or had diarrhoea? Have you noticed blood in your stools? These are just some of the questions you might ask.

TIP: When a patient points out the location of their pain, visualise the tissues that may be causing the pain and the systems or organs that can refer pain to that location. These are the systems to focus on in your systemic review.

The following are some examples of the types of questions you might ask relating to each system. Remember – you must find your own words to use which you are comfortable with, and which fit your particular style.

Cardiovascular system

- Any chest pain? Or pain to the arm, neck or face?

- Are you ever short of breath when you would not expect to be?

- Are you ever particularly aware of your heartbeat?

- Do you get swollen hands and feet?

- Do you ever feel faint or light headed?

- Do you have piles or varicose veins?

Respiratory system

- Any chest pain?

- Do you have a cough?

- When you cough, do you bring anything up?
  (colour, blood?)

- Are you ever short of breath when you would not expect to be?

- Is your breathing wheezy?

Gastrointestinal system

- Is your weight changing or stable?
  (Clothes tight / loose)

- Do you have any problems or change to your bowel habit?

- Do you have any pain in your abdomen?

- Do you suffer from heartburn or indigestion?

- Do you feel nauseous or do you vomit?

- Do you suffer from wind particularly?

Genitourinary system

- Any problems with, or change to your bladder habit?

- Any pain passing water?

- Any problems starting or stopping? (Men)

- Any incontinence?

- How many times do you get up in the night to pass water?

- Do you ever see blood or pus in your urine?

Genitourinary system – Sexual function

- Has there been any change in your libido or sex drive?

- Do you experience any erectile dysfunction?

- Do have pain on intercourse?

Please be aware, these are extremely intimate questions, and as such, you will need to have clear clinical justification for asking them, and you will need to explain to the patient your reasoning.

Gynaecological system

- Any problems or change with your periods?

- Are your periods regular?

- When was your last period?

- Do you have any bleeding between periods?

- Do you have any discharge?

- Have you had your menopause?

- Are you on HRT?

- Do you have any children? If so, how many?

- Do you have regular smear tests?

Nervous system

- Are you in pain?

- Do you suffer from headaches?

- Any blurred or double vision?

- Ever suffered from episodes of fainting, fits or blackouts?

- Do you have ringing in your ears, deafness or dizziness?

- Do you experience numbness or tingling in your arms or legs?

- Any weakness or stiffness in your limbs?

- Have you noticed any changes in your coordination?

- Do you feel depressed or tense, or suffer from anxiety?

Many students struggle with questioning their patients regarding their systemic health. They are unsure which questions to ask, and how many. How do you know when to stop questioning? I know some practitioners dread their patient saying 'Yes' to a question because they are not sure where to take it from there.

Remember, we are trying to assess the patient's systemic health to understand how it relates to their presenting complaint, but just as importantly, if the patient has signs of a systemic problem, we need to know how urgent and how serious it is, because we need to be able to decide what action (if any) we should take. Do we need to call an ambulance for them? Do we need to write a letter to their doctor? Do we need to reassure the patient, but advise they speak to their doctor at some time? Do we just note their symptoms and monitor them? We don't necessarily need to form a definitive diagnosis of their systemic condition, but we need to have a good idea of what's wrong, and which system is affected, and what action (if any) needs to be taken. Let me give an example from my own practice.

My patient is a 70-year-old retired plumber. He complains of generalised low back pain with no neurological signs or symptoms to his legs. He's very stiff in the morning for half an hour or so, and is stiff in all movements of his back. My systemic enquiry went something like this:

'How's your health in general?'
'I think it's pretty good thanks.'
'Any ongoing medical conditions you are aware of?'
'No, I'm all good.'
'Any problems or change to your bowel habit?'
'No, I'm pretty regular.'
'Any problems or change to your bladder habit?'
'Not really, I'm just getting older.'
'Do you feel that's affected your bladder habit then?'
'Well, us men all get a bit slower as we get older eh?'
'I know what you mean. Do you feel that your flow of urine has reduced then?'
'Well as I say, it's normal for my age eh?'

'Well it's certainly quite common. Do you have any problem starting to have a pee?'

'Yes, it does take a while sometimes. I might stand at the toilet for a few seconds before it kicks in.'

'And once you are peeing, do you have any trouble stopping?'

'No, that's fine.'

'Any leaks?'

'No, thank goodness.'

'Do you think you're peeing more often than you used to?'

'Yes, I think so.'

'Do you have to get up in the night to have a pee?'

'Yes, I do. I'm usually up a couple of times in the night.'

'So you're peeing more frequently than you used to. Volume-wise, are you peeing little and often, or peeing a lot and often?

'No, not much each time, but more often.'

'How long have you been noticing these changes?'

'Oh, probably over the past couple of years or so.'

'Have these symptom been getting worse?'

'Not really.'

'Have you noticed any blood in your urine?'

'No, not at all.'

'Have you spoken to your doctor about this?'

'No, I don't like to bother her, she's very busy.'

I then went on to ask questions like: Any chest pain? Are you ever short of breath when you wouldn't expect to be? Any regular cough? Are you a headachy person? Is your weight changing or stable? How are your energy levels? My patient said no to everything.

What are your thoughts?

My thinking was that this gentleman is of an age at which his prostate may give problems, so I would generally ask some prostate-specific questions even if he'd answered no to 'any problems or change to your bladder habit'. But he answered 'not really, just getting older', and then further questioning confirmed issues.

So, what do we do?

In this case, he may well have benign prostate hypertrophy. It's not a medical emergency – it's been going on for some time, and not getting much worse. Although he reports no blood in his urine, we can't rule out prostate cancer. We could get into a discussion of the likelihood of his back pain being related to his prostate problems. If he has prostate cancer, it could have metastasized to his back and/or pelvis, or does he just have benign hypertrophy and degenerative changes to his lumbar spine related to his age and work history? His responses to our questions relating to his presenting complaint would help us decide.

How would you manage this patient?

In this case I had a conversation with him along the lines of 'you're right, some men do find their flow a bit reduced as they get older due to their prostate getting a little enlarged. This isn't a serious medical condition, but I think it's important for you to discuss the situation with your doctor, who will probably suggest some tests to find out exactly what is going on. I can help by writing a letter for you to take to the doctor explaining why I've advised you to consult them. Would you like me to do this?' In the case of this gentleman, he was a little reluctant, saying she's very busy', so I then said 'Would you feel more comfortable discussing this with a male doctor?' To which he replied 'Yes, I think I would. It's a bit embarrassing.' So I said I'd look up which other doctors worked at his GP's practice, and would write to a male doctor and he should make an appointment to talk to them soon.

As a side note: often the key thing we are looking for is a *change* in something. If we take bowel habits for example, one person may open their bowels three or four times a day, and another every second day. If they have always been like this, then this is their normal. If the person who usually defecates every other day starts going twice a day, then this would be a concern. It's outside their normal habit.

Another side note: many of the questions we ask are of a personal nature. You must practice asking these questions so that you become relaxed and confident. If you are hesitant, or appear awkward and embarrassed, the patient will also feel embarrassed.

Remember:

- When carrying out a systemic enquiry, you do not just tick yes or no to your questions. You must follow up all positive responses until you have enough information to make an assessment and develop a plan of action.
- You have to decide which questions to ask or not ask based on the case in hand, and you must be able to justify your decisions.
- Practice asking questions in everyday language. Your patient may not understand technical or medical terms.

Red flags

Red flags are aspects of the case history that alert you to the possibility that your patient may have a condition that requires referral to a doctor for medical attention, or a condition that if not investigated or treated would be detrimental to the patient's general wellbeing. The seriousness and nature of the suspected condition will determine what action you take, and the degree of urgency required. Some practitioners talk of 'total' red flags: conditions that require immediate referral and treatment, and 'partial' red flags: conditions that require investigation in the near future. If in doubt, err on the side of caution!

There is no definitive list of red flags; however, suspect red flag pathology if your patient complains of any of the following:

- Severe unremitting pain.

- Deep constant ache or throbbing.

- Severe night pain.

- Severe pain with no history of trauma or injury.

- Constant pain unaffected by medication or position.

- Unusual protective posture.

- Bizarre symptom picture.

- Fever, unexplained weight loss, generalised weakness, pallor or jaundice.

This list is by no means exhaustive. Use your knowledge of pathology to decide if a patient is safe to examine, and/or treat, or if they are reporting or displaying signs or symptoms of pathology requiring referral.

Other flags

When I was a student, I'm sure there were only red flags, but over time, the flag system has got a whole lot more colourful. We now have yellow flags for psychosocial risk factors, orange flags which are similar to red flags but for mental health issues, black flags for occupational factors, and blue flags which relate to an individual's perception about work and their health.

Safeguarding

By building a professional therapeutic relationship with our patients, we allow them to feel safe and comfortable in the clinical setting. Patients know we are bound by confidentiality guidelines and they often feel able to talk to us about anything, which may lead to disclosures of a safeguarding nature. During our examination, we will see the physical manifestations of their life experiences. You will be surprised by some of the information your patients will share with you, and with some of the physical injuries you may see. You may come across cases of abuse or domestic violence, for example. Handling these patients requires a high level of skill and training. You will receive some training in this area as part of your undergraduate programme, and it is your responsibility to remain updated with current laws and regulations as part of your CPD. Safeguarding training is available through your Local Authority Safeguarding Board, who will be happy to advise you on all aspects of safeguarding adults and children. Please investigate what is available to help you as a practitioner, and familiarise yourself with the resources available in your area to support victims of abuse.

Fifty common diseases

In an ideal world, we would be familiar with the signs and symptoms of all pathologies and the 'profile' of those people most likely to suffer from them. In time, you may well gather this mass of knowledge, but as a student, the sheer size of the subject can make its study seem overwhelming. So, I have a suggestion: Below is a list of 50 common diseases (actually, there are 59, but 50 makes for a snappier title). I would suggest that this is a good starting point, and a very manageable task. Why not agree a plan with yourself to take, say, five diseases each week. For each one, learn the signs and symptoms of the pathology. What will the patient look like? How will they describe their problem? Also, what would be the typical age and sex of the patient? What questions would you use to investigate the problem? This list will probably cover 99% of the pathologies you'll see in clinic.

CVS	Myocardial infarction
	Angina
	Hypertension
	Peripheral vascular disease
Respiratory	Asthma
	Acute / chronic bronchitis
	Pneumonia
	Cancer of the lung

Abdomen	Stomach / duodenal ulcers
	Cancer of the colon
	Gallstones
	Hernias
	Haemorrhoids
	Appendicitis
	Hepatitis
Nervous system	Meningitis
	Epilepsy
	Parkinson's
	CVA and intra-cranial bleed
	Headache syndromes
Endocrine system	Thyroid disease
	Diabetes
	Cushing's
Musculoskeletal	Rheumatoid arthritis
	Osteoarthritis
	Systemic lupus eryethematosus.
	Polymyalgia rheumatica (PMR)
	Ankylosing spondylitis
	Fibromyalgia
Psychiatric	Depression
	Anxiety
	Psychoses
	Schizophrenia
Genitourinary	Urinary tract infection / cystitis
	Kidney stones
	Benign / malignant prostate
Skin	Eczema
	Psoriasis
	Urticaria
ENT	Otitis media
	Tonsillitis
	Meniere's disease

Reproductive	Menstrual disturbance
	Infertility
	Chlamydia
	Syphilis
	Gonorrhea
	AIDS
Eyes	Conjunctivitis
	Cataracts
	Glaucoma
	Iritis
Childhood	Childhood exanthema
	Developmental problems
Geriatrics	Incontinence
	Mental deterioration
Miscellaneous	Shingles
	Malaria
	TB

TIP: When researching these diseases, a good place to start is the NHS website *nhs.uk/conditions/*. It contains easy to understand basic information about many conditions. Start here, and if you then want more in-depth knowledge, move on to your pathology books.

ANOTHER TIP: if you have a patient who has a pathology of some sort, or even a friend or family member, ask them all about it. If it's a patient, let's say they have Parkinson's, maybe while you're treating them, you could say something like; 'Do you mind telling me about your Parkinson's?' Find out what they first noticed. What symptoms do they have? How old were they when they first thought something wasn't right? How did it get diagnosed? How has it progressed? How does it affect their day-to-day life? And then, that very day, look up Parkinson's and check how the description in your books or online compares to your patient's story. You'll remember everything about it then because you have a real patient to hang the knowledge on.

Past medical history

We need to ask our patients about their past medical history for several reasons:

- Safety: Their past health may contraindicate certain examinations or techniques.
- There may be a direct link to the patient's presenting complaint. A past illness, accident or operation may have predisposed them to today's problem.
- Today's problem may be a progression of an earlier problem.
- Their past health may give an insight into their ability to recover from injury and illness.

We generally question patients about their past medical history in three areas:

1. Have they had any significant accidents or sporting injuries?
2. Have they had any serious illnesses?
3. Have they had any operations?

These three questions will cover most eventualities. However, it's a good idea to start with a general question such as: 'Generally, how has your health been in the past?'

Note: All positive responses need to be followed up. If they have had a road traffic accident, for example, what happened? When was it? Were they injured? Did they have to go to hospital? The same goes for operations: what was it for? Was it successful? When was it? Etc. When it comes to past illnesses, I avoid asking 'Have you ever been ill?' because everyone has been ill at some time in their life. I generally ask something like 'Have you ever had any significant illnesses, other than minor childhood illnesses?'

Are there any medical conditions that seem to run in your patient's family? If so, could your patient have the same condition? How relevant is it to their presenting complaint and their health in general? Do your patient's symptoms suggest a hereditary condition? A family history of the condition will add weight to your hypothesis.

When investigating a patient's family history, I tend to ask something like 'Are there any conditions that seem to run in your family?' I word it like this, because generally, we're not interested in knowing about the health of every family member past and present. This can eat up time. We are interested in anything that seems to be a common factor in the patient's family health.

Social history

We are trying to build a 'big picture' of what is wrong with our patient, what caused their present problem, what predisposed them to injury or dysfunction and what is maintaining their problem – the global picture. Information regarding your patient's social situation forms an important part of their case history.

- What does their work involve? Physical demands and stress may be factors.
- What is their home situation? You need to be cautious when asking for information such as whether they live alone, do they have children and marital status etc. However, it can be useful to understand the demands on them at home and whether there is anyone to support them while they are incapacitated, for example.
- What, if any, exercise do they take? This may give an insight into their general health, their likelihood to respond to treatment, or indeed, may be a causative factor.

Note that some areas of questioning, in some circumstances, do not need to be asked at the initial consultation (or may never be asked if you do not feel the information is relevant to the patient's situation). As you build a relationship with your patient, you can gather more information to fill in any gaps as appropriate. If a patient responds to a question with 'Why do you need to know that?' it's important that you can give a good, clear clinical reason.

As a side point: I sometimes give an explanation before the question is raised. For instance, if I have a patient with low back pain, I will ask early on if the pain is only in their back, or if the pain is in their legs as well, and if they have any problems or change to their bowels, bladder and periods since the injury. Some patients may not understand why they are being asked what seem like quite personal questions. So immediately after asking, I might say something like 'I ask because the nerves from your lower back supply the area where you have pain, but they also have branches which supply your legs and some internal organs, so this information can be very helpful.'

Diet

What relevance does your patient's diet have to you as a practitioner? Well:

- Poor diet can lead to poor healing. This may be a factor to consider when developing a prognosis.
- Your patient's diet may be directly linked to the problem they are consulting you about. A gastrointestinal problem for example.

For each case, you must ask yourself: how relevant is your patient's diet to their presenting complaint and to their health in general? This will determine the range and depth of questioning appropriate for this patient.

TIP: Asking a question like: 'Do you eat a balanced diet' usually requires a number of follow-up questions and often fails to elicit objective information. If you feel that diet is not a significant factor in a patient's case, you may simply ask: 'are you on any special diet?' If you feel that you need more information, you could ask: 'Tell me what you ate yesterday?' This will give a good objective snapshot. For a full breakdown, ask the patient to complete a food diary over the coming week. Remember though: you decide what to ask based on the case in hand. Time spent asking unnecessary questions is time wasted.

Allergies

We need to know if the patient is allergic to anything. They may be sensitive to something you may use during the treatment – creams or oils for example. In addition, the range and severity of the patient's allergies may give an insight into how reactive they might be to certain techniques. In general, if a patient has a wide range of allergies and sensitivities, I tend to treat them more gently.

Impact

I feel it's good practice to ask the patient how their present injury or health issue impacts their daily life. Does it stop them doing anything in particular? Can they care for themselves? Does it stop them working, or make their work difficult? Understanding the affect their health is having on their life doesn't directly help us work out what is wrong with them, but it helps us to build an effective therapeutic relationship with the patient, and allows us to show empathy. In addition, as the patient recovers, we can track the improvements relative to the patient's abilities to do more in their day-to-day life.

Expectations

Your patient will have certain expectations prior to seeing you. It's important to understand what they are, early on during the session. I may simply ask 'what are your expectations from your visit here today?' Your patient may be expecting to be completely pain free after one session, or they may be expecting x-ray investigations, or health and exercise advice for example. Have a discussion with them, and start to manage their expectations. If they are expecting something which they don't get, or is unrealistic, they may well be dissatisfied.

Inhibitors to effective case history taking

Over the 25 years that I've been working in a teaching clinic, I've seen many students take a first-class history. They've developed a good rapport with their patient; listened well and got all the information needed to fully understand the patient's condition and circumstances. The patient has felt listened to, and been understood. Sometimes, particularly in the early days of being a student practitioner, it has gone less well. I always encourage my students to be honest with themselves, and reflect on the session and pick out the good and the not so good elements. (By the way, all experienced practitioners should do this all the time too.) We mustn't be hard on ourselves, but instead identify how it could have gone better, and feel positive that the next time it *will* be better.

Most times when a case history has been taken poorly, it's due to one or more of three reasons:

- Poor communication.
- Poor background knowledge.
- Lack of practice.

Communication

Remember this principle: the key to effective osteopathy is communication.

The only way to be effective as a practitioner is by communicating at the highest level with the patient; both physically in terms of examination and treatment, and non-physically in terms of verbal interaction and body language.

If you cannot communicate with your patient, how can you gather the information you need to treat them? Poor communication leads to poor diagnosis which leads to poor treatment (and an unsuccessful career). Good communication skills will enable you to build relationships with your patients. You will then gather all the information you need to manage their healthcare effectively. In doing so, they will value your work and recommend you to others – which is good for your patients and good for your business! Some people are naturally good communicators – it's a quality they have. Others are less gifted, so they need to work hard to acquire this skill, and they need to practise over and over until it comes naturally. Reflect on how good you are at communicating effectively, and take action as required.

Knowledge

I posed the question earlier: if an elephant entered the room, how would you know it's an elephant?' I used it to explain how we need background knowledge of musculoskeletal conditions and medical conditions in order to recognise them when a patient tells us their story. You can never have too much knowledge, and we should never stop learning. We also need to be good at applying our knowledge in a clinical setting.

How can you identify the tissue causing pain if you are not familiar with the relative anatomical structures and the types of pain they produce? How will you know if your patient is suffering from, say, bowel cancer if you do not know about bowel cancer – who gets it, common age of onset, signs and symptoms etc? Without a good knowledge of pathology and physiology you may be unsafe. How can you develop a hypothesis including aetiological factors and maintaining factors without knowledge of body mechanics and function? How can you form a picture of your patient's global health situation without real depth of knowledge? It is in the consulting room where everything you have learned is drawn upon to enable you to be a competent, safe and successful practitioner.

Be honest with yourself, identify your strengths and weaknesses, and feel good about making plans to be the best practitioner you can be.

We need excellent communication skills in order to apply our knowledge effectively. The only way to achieve this is with constant practice. Practice doesn't have to be in a clinical setting. Friends and family will have health issues from time to time. Ask them if you can take their history. The more practice you get, the more confident you will become, and patients respond better to confident practitioners.

Remember, there is a finite time available to take the history, examine the patient, form a diagnosis and treat the patient. Time spent taking a good case history is well spent. If you are clear and logical in your interviewing, able to think on your feet, and adapt your questioning as appropriate, you will quickly have all the facts. This will allow more time for examination and treatment.

Remember:

- It takes less time to take a case history well, than to take one badly.
- Time wasted during poor history taking is time lost examining and treating your patients.

There are many ways to take a case history. The method I have described here is one that has served me well throughout many years in practice. I urge you to explore and research other methods and formats, and develop a style that suits you. Whether you are a student, or an experienced practitioner, if someone suggests a particular way you should take a history, ask them to justify their way, and take from it the parts that will help you to become the best that you can be.

Work hard. Communicate well. Enjoy every patient interaction. Be fabulous!

Questioning

Life provides us all with the qualities and skills required to take a case history. After all, it's just a conversation; but not just any conversation – a very important conversation – a structured conversation, a conversation that will gather all the facts required for us to form a plan of examination and diagnosis.

In order to gather the facts, we must ask questions and understand the responses, we must communicate effectively. This means asking questions in a way that will encourage the patient to give us the relevant information, but not to overload us with spurious or irrelevant information. (It may be very interesting to hear a blow-by-blow account of the patient's recent holiday but how helpful is it to you?)

There is a fine line between making your patient feel comfortable enough to answer your questions fully, and having them dominate the session with irrelevant information. The skilful use of different types of questions will allow you to gather the information you require effectively, in a friendly, professional way.

Open questions

These are questions such as: 'What is the problem you have come about today?' and 'What does your work involve?' Open questions encourage the patient to talk openly and can elicit a lot of information. They cannot be answered with a simple yes or no. On the downside, the patient may start to ramble and impart too much, or irrelevant information. On occasion, it is difficult to note down replies to open questions.

Closed questions

These are questions such as 'Is the pain sharp?' or 'How many children do you have?' They cause the patient to give a short, precise answer – often yes or no. Closed questions can be used to good effect when clarifying information and for gaining precise information. They allow you as a practitioner a high level of control, and are easy to note. However, too many closed questions can make the interview less of a conversation and more of an interrogation.

Menu questions

These are useful when you need precise information and your patient is maybe a little slow or unclear with their responses. For example, you may ask, 'How would you describe your pain?' If the patient replies 'It's an ache' then fine. If they hesitate, or cannot seem to find the right words, you might ask: 'For example, is the pain sharp, aching or burning?' while you do not want to lead the patient, you need to get the information within a reasonable time.

Note: menu questions list a number of related options which encourage the patient to pick one as an answer. Menu questions are not the same as multiple questions. Multiple questions are questions such as 'Have you had any shortness of breath, headaches, heartburn, fever etc?' Questions like this lead to confusion and often require clarification.

A skilful practitioner will intermix different types of questions to quickly elicit the information required while maintaining a professional, friendly rapport. The ability to do this will develop with practice.

Confirmation, clarification, confrontation

Confirmation, clarification and confrontation are useful techniques to ensure you have accurately understood what the patient is telling you. Hearing the information is one thing, understanding the information is something else!

Confirmation is where you reflect back to the patient what you have understood. It gives the patient an opportunity to correct any misunderstanding and confirms to the patient that you are following their story. For example: 'So, if I understand you correctly, when you lifted the box yesterday, you felt a twinge in your back, but this morning you woke with severe pain?'

Clarification builds on the information already gathered. For example: 'You say the pain came on the day after you lifted the box; when exactly?'

Confrontation is something many of us try to avoid in daily life. However, in this instance it is not used in a negative way. Confrontation is used to gently clarify the facts when there appears to be conflicting details. For example: 'I think I may have misheard you – did you say that you are unable to walk more than a few steps since your injury, yet you have continued to go to work?'

Never be embarrassed to ask the patient to clarify a point, or repeat what they have said, or to expand on the information they have given you. As long as your patient understands why you need the information, they will draw comfort and confidence from the fact that you are obviously keen to understand fully their problem and circumstances.

Osteopathic sieve

The osteopathic sieve is a concept developed by the osteopath Audrey Smith in the late 1960s. It is based on the fact that pathological processes fall into a number of classes, and that these processes occur in 'families' of tissues.

A full explanation of the osteopathic sieve is outside the scope of this book. I mention it though, because I have adopted and adapted some of the classifications used in the sieve for use as a learning aid, and as an aid to differential diagnosis.

The sieve as a learning tool: Generate a file or page for each body region: head, neck, shoulders, elbows, wrists, hands, thoracic spine, lumbar spine, pelvis, hips, knees and ankles. Then for each region, divide it into sections labelled as per the sieve categories: congenital, infectious, inflammatory, neoplastic, traumatic, degenerative, referred, vascular, functional and metabolic. For each region, research and list all the conditions and pathologies that can affect that area for each category. For example: on the lumbar spine page, under congenital, we might list spondylolysthesis, sacrelised lumbar vertebra, lumberised sacrum, spina bifida etc. For each condition, research and list things like: who gets it? What age? What sex? What are the signs and symptoms? How would the patient describe it? How is it diagnosed? What differentiates it from other conditions?

The sieve as an aid to differential diagnosis: Occasionally, our reasoning can become blinkered. We may think we know what the problem is early on in the interview, and miss other likely causes of the patient's symptoms. We may inadvertently ask questions to confirm our theory, rather than asking questions to explore all possibilities. After taking the case history of a new patient, take a few minutes to consider their symptoms against each of the above sieve categories. As a student, after taking the case history, you might say to the patient something like, 'Please let me just take a minute to review my notes to make sure I've got all the information I need.' And then in your head, run through the sieve categories. In the case of low back pain for example, you might be thinking that the patient has a disc injury. But just consider, could this person's pain be due to a congenital problem? Could it be due to an inflammatory or infective condition? And so on. In each case, you will be drawing on the knowledge of the conditions in each category, and comparing them to the patient's presentation. You may suddenly consider the possibility of another cause, and ask further questions to test this possibility. Even if you cannot identify the exact condition, you may well be able to decide which category it is in, and still be able to manage the situation.

Note taking

As stated at the start of this guide, to be able to take a case history efficiently requires a range of skills and qualities. You must be able to communicate effectively with your patient to build a rapport such that you can gather all the facts and information necessary to formulate an examination plan. Based on the information gathered during the interview and examination, and by drawing on your knowledge of pathology, physiology, body mechanics etc, you will form an assessment or diagnosis. Based on this, you will agree and implement, with the patient, a treatment and management plan. Throughout all of this you must take notes!

Take time to note the following general points regarding your notes:

- The notes should be written contemporaneously (at the time of the interview).
- Write clearly and legibly preferably using dark ink. (The notes may need to be copied)
- Your patient has a right to look at the notes or ask for a copy. DO NOT write anything in them that you would not like the patient to see.
- The notes for your patient are your responsibility. Should there be a problem, the buck stops with you

- In the UK, the Data Protection Act 2018 controls how personal information is used by organisations, businesses or the government.
  The Data Protection Act 2018 is the UK's implementation of the General Data Protection Regulation (GDPR). Everyone responsible for using personal data has to follow strict rules called 'data protection principles'. As osteopaths, your notes form part of a patient's health record, and you must therefore ensure you adhere to GDPR regulations. The Information Commissioner's Office (ICO) is very helpful in guiding you through your legal responsibilities in this area.

In most practices, pre-printed case notes are used. The various sections are filled in as the interview progresses. Let me repeat my earlier statement: Your questioning should not follow a rigid format or order. There is a logical way or system of working through each case, but each case will be different, and will require you to think on your feet and question as appropriate.

Most history files have two main parts:

1. The part completed when the patient presents as a new patient. This will detail the information gathered regarding the presenting complaint, past medical history, general health, your initial examination findings, your diagnosis, and your treatment and management plans.

2. The continuation sheets. On every visit, you must note how the patient has progressed since the last treatment, today's examination findings, today's diagnosis and today's treatment and advice. Remember SOAP?

There is a real art to taking good notes while taking a case history, and it only comes with practice. For effective case history taking we really do need a 'multi-tasking brain.' The difficulty lies in that we are required to do several things at the same time: we are developing a picture of what may be wrong with the patient based on the information they are giving us. We are then using this information to decide what to ask next and so refine our differential diagnosis. While this is going on, we must demonstrate good listening skills such as maintaining appropriate eye contact, body language etc. Throughout the whole time we must write appropriate notes. Long silences while you slowly write down every word break the flow of the interview. Once you have the patient at ease and telling their story, you must maintain that rapport and flow. In physical therapy, there are many common abbreviations. It is vital you get used to using these. With practice, the art of talking, listening, thinking and writing at the same time will come to you. Note that I said 'with practice'!

TIP: Although the notes may be pre-printed, you do not have to complete each section in order. If for example, while investigating a presenting complaint of Low Back Pain, the patient mentions their concerns regarding some systemic problem, it may be reassuring to the patient to cover this area now and come back to the presenting complaint. In this case, note the systemic information in the appropriate part of the form.

ANOTHER TIP: There are occasions when systemic information should be included with the presenting complaint. If for example, a patient complains of low back pain. You would obviously ask about radiations, parasthesia, and problems or change to bowel and bladder function (associated symptoms). If they report, say, constipation which seems to relate to the onset of low back pain, then I would argue that this information should be recorded along with the presenting complaint, as well as under the systemic enquiry heading.

Examination plan and findings

Let's assume you have taken the case history. You started by visualising the area of pain, you asked intelligent questions to build up a picture of the tissues that might be involved, you have run through your osteopathic sieve and formulated a list of possible diagnoses (your differential diagnosis). If you have taken the history well, you will have already narrowed down the number of possibilities to maybe two or three. Now you must test your hypotheses. You must construct an examination plan that will effectively and efficiently rule in or out the various possibilities; such that you can arrive at your diagnosis or assessment.

Remember, too little examination and testing may lead to misdiagnosis and may be dangerous; too much examination is inefficient and wastes time. You must be able to justify the examinations that you chose to undertake or not undertake.

Diagnosis

Over the years, I have seen many students struggle when it comes to formulating the words to describe their diagnosis. They have taken a good case history, devised and conducted an excellent examination, and formulated an impressive treatment and management plan. They absolutely 'know' what is wrong with the patient, and what needs to be done, but then struggle to put their assessment into words to write in the notes in the diagnosis box.

As is the case with many aspects of history taking, there is no set format for writing a diagnosis. It is good practice, however, if your diagnosis includes the following information:

- Tissue causing pain:
  This may be something like 'left anterior cruciate ligament sprain' or 'osteoarthritis of the right hip with associated muscle contracture' or 'somatic dysfunction of the L/S junction'.
- Aetiology:
  In other words, what caused the injury? It may be something like: 'traumatic fall while skiing', or 'road traffic accident', or 'laying paving slabs'.
- Predisposing factors:
  These are the factors which enabled the injury to occur. Factors such as 'repetitive use of a keyboard', or 'primary

short lower extremity (PSLE)' or 'chronically restricted thoracic spine' or 'recent childbirth'.

- Maintaining factors:
  These are the factors which hinder the patient's recovery.
  For example: 'occupation (sitting at work station for long
  periods)', 'looking after a baby' or 'failure to rest post injury'.

By including the above factors in our diagnosis, our assessment
becomes more 'osteopathic' and holistic. Some of the factors may
blur, or be the same, but on the whole, a clearer picture of what
has happened to the patient, why it has happened and why they
have not got better will emerge.

Example:

Your patient has developed left groin and buttock pain during a
recent walking holiday. He is a 67-year-old retired postman. He had
a similar episode a year ago. His GP referred him for x-ray investigation which revealed osteoarthritis of the left hip.

This may seem quite black and white – your diagnosis may be 'Osteoarthritis of the left hip'. However, we can improve on this. Sup-
pose there is pain due to a protective contracture of the left glutes
and piriformis? We could then expand our diagnosis to 'Pain due to
osteoarthritis of the left hip with associated contracture of the left
gluteal and piriformis muscles.'

This builds a better picture. But what led to this problem? You may
find he has a long left leg. Also, why have his symptoms suddenly
appeared? What about the walking holiday?

So, now we may say our patient has 'Pain due to osteoarthritis of
the left hip with associated contracture of the left gluteal and
piriformis muscles, aggravated by a recent walking holiday, predisposed and maintained by a PSLE.' This builds a real picture of what
is happening with this patient.

In fact, there may be more: we may discover his partner passed
away last year, and he has been struggling to care for himself. We
can weave into our assessment components like poor diet and

mental health factors. By acknowledging all the various factors that have led to your patient's present health situation, you can develop a plan to address each aspect. This is holistic healthcare.

Management plan

Here is the detail of how you intend to manage your patient. Often, practitioners find it logical to split this into short-term and long-term plans.

Your short-term plan may include:

- The treatment you intend to do today and over the coming few weeks.
- Advice you intend to give the patient, for example: 'Advised patient to apply hot/cold three times/day for 15 minutes.'
- Any action you plan. For example: 'Will refer to GP if BP stays high over next two treatments.'

Your long-term plan should detail what you intend to achieve over the coming months or possibly years. For example: 'Implement a monthly or quarterly treatment plan to prevent recurrence of recent injury.'

The final word

I hope you find this short guide useful in your preparation for clinic and practice life. My final words repeat some of my earlier advice:

Case history taking is not a fixed, rigid process. It involves human interaction and as such should be fluid. I suggest you use the format outlined in this guide; however, you must think on your feet, constantly changing and adapting your questioning as the case unfolds.

Of course, as you gain experience, you will find your own way of taking a case history. As long as it's effective and conforms to the guidance of your governing professional body, then go ahead. What I've outlined here though, is a good place to start.

Remember the inhibitors to effective case history taking: poor communication skills, poor knowledge and lack of practice. All of these things are in your control. Constantly review the knowledge you gain elsewhere in your training; your pathology, anatomy, neurology, etc. and bring it to good use in the consulting room. And don't forget the osteopathy!

Practice is the only way to become efficient at case history taking. Don't wait until your final exams to find out your weaknesses.

Remember that taking the history is a conversation. Relax and enjoy it!

Personal reflection

From time to time while writing this book, I have reflected on exactly why I'm doing it. After all, although it's quite a short book, it's taken quite a bit of work to put together. Well, it's not for the money – it's not likely to make the *Sunday Times Best Seller list* is it? And it's not for any egotistical reasons either.

I've written this book to help you.

If you're a student, I hope it will give you the knowledge, inspiration and confidence to become the best that you can be. If you are already a practitioner, I hope you have found something in this book to enhance your practice, and help you get the most out of your working day.

Please let me know if this book has helped you, and if so, in what way? I would also love to have your suggestions on how the book could be improved.

Terry Rulten

Email me at: osteoterry@gmail.com